COOKIES OR CARROTS?

YOU ARE WHAT YOU EAT

OBESITY & KIDS

COOKIES OR CARROTS?

YOU ARE WHAT YOU EAT

BY HELEN THOMPSON

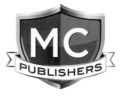

Mason Crest Publishers

MASON CREST PUBLISHERS INC.
370 Reed Road
Broomall, Pennsylvania 19008
(866)MCP-BOOK (toll free)
www.masoncrest.com

First Printing
9 8 7 6 5 4 3 2 1

          Library of Congress Cataloging-in-Publication Data

Thompson, Helen.
 Cookies or carrots? you are what you eat / by Helen Thompson.
     p. cm.
 Includes bibliographical references and index.
 ISBN 978-1-4222-1707-8   ISBN 978-1-4222-1705-4 (series)
 ISBN 978-1-4222-1895-2 (pbk.)   ISBN 978-1-4222-1893-8 (pbk. series)
 1. Nutrition—Juvenile literature. I. Title.
 RA784.T528 2010
 613.2—dc22
                        2010025502

Design by MK Bassett-Harvey.
Produced by Harding House Publishing Service, Inc.
www.hardinghousepages.com
Cover design by Torque Advertising and Design.
Printed in USA by Bang Printing.

CONTENTS

INTRODUCTION
FOR THE TEACHERS

We as a society often reserve our harshest criticism for those conditions we understand the least. Such is the case for obesity. Obesity is a chronic and often-fatal disease that accounts for 400,000 deaths each year. It is second only to smoking as a cause of premature death in the United States. People suffering from obesity need understanding, support, and medical assistance. Yet what they often receive is scorn.

Today, children are the fastest growing segment of the obese population in the United States. This constitutes a public health crisis of enormous proportions. Living with childhood obesity affects self-esteem, which down the road can affect employment and attainment of higher education. But childhood obesity is much more than a social stigma. It has serious health consequences.

Childhood obesity increases the risk for poor health in adulthood—but also even during childhood. Depression, diabetes, asthma, gallstones, orthopedic diseases, and other obesity-related conditions are all on the rise in children. Recent estimates suggest that 30 to 50 percent of children born in 2000 will develop type 2 diabetes mellitus, a leading cause of preventable blindness, kidney failure, heart disease, stroke, and amputations. Obesity is undoubtedly the most pressing nutritional disorder among young people today.

If we are to reverse obesity's current trend, there must be family, community, and national objectives promoting healthy eating and exercise. As a nation, we must demand broad-based public-health initiatives to limit TV watching, curtail junk food advertising toward children, and promote physical activity. More than rhetoric, these need to be our rallying cry. Anything short of this will eventually fail, and within our lifetime obesity will become the leading cause of death in the United States if not in the world. This series is an excellent first step in battling the obesity crisis by educating young children about the risks, the realities, and what they can do to build healthy lifestyles right now.

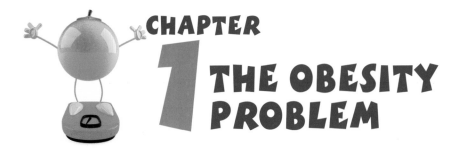

CHAPTER 1
THE OBESITY PROBLEM

The people of the world are getting heavier. Even while people are starving in some areas of the world, in other places, more and more people are overweight and obese. In the past, only the richest nations (like the United States) had this problem, but more and more today, even poorer nations are facing the problem of *obesity*. This is partly because cheap foods—fast foods, sweet foods, and starchy foods—are often also the foods that are most likely to make you fat!

"Obese" is the word doctors use when someone is seriously overweight. Although being overweight isn't as dangerous to your health as being obese, doctors and scientists have

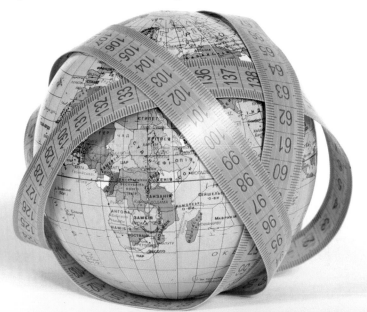

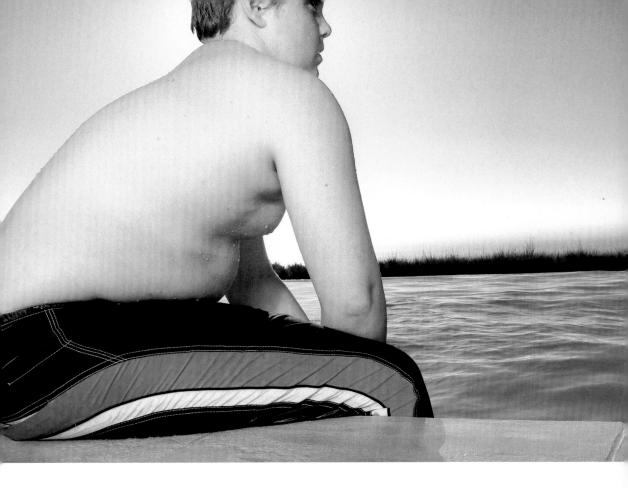

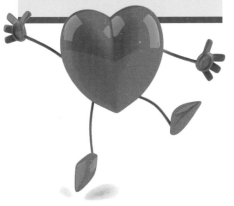

Obesity is when a person has so much extra body fat that it's a danger to health.

found that even being a little too fat can make a person more likely to get sick. Heart disease, diabetes, arthritis, and some kinds of cancer can all be caused by being overweight or obese. And it's not just adults who face these dangers. Children can be at risk too.

So what caused all this? Why are so many people fat?

WHY ARE PEOPLE SO FAT?

Many of your grandparents and their grandparents grew their own food. They cooked their own food. And they saved food for the winter by canning or drying it. Food took up a lot of people's time.

Today all that has changed. Most people no longer grow their food. Instead, people buy it at grocery stores. Lots of people

DID YOU KNOW?

According to the World Health Organization, at least 400 million adults around the world are obese, and another 1.6 billion are overweight. At least 20 million children under 5 are also overweight.

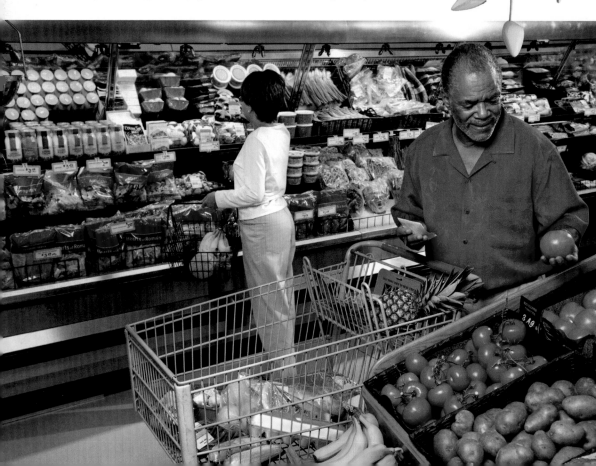

don't eat at home. They don't always have time to cook. Life moves faster than it once did too. Many people drive cars. These cars are produced in factories—and so is our food. Food production has become a big business. Whether we make our food at home or eat out at restaurants, most people want their food produced as quickly and cheaply as possible. And we learned to believe that BIGGER and MORE are always better.

What does **global** mean?

It means that something is found all around the world.

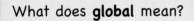

FAST FOOD

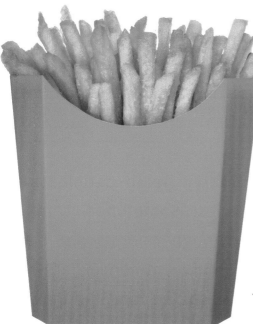

You probably take for granted that fast-food restaurants are on nearly every city block. Today, MacDonalds restaurants have gone *global.*

But it wasn't always that way. Fast-food restaurants didn't exist until the mid-twentieth century. Once they started, though, they caught on quickly. Before long, many kinds of food were being made as fast foods, from hamburgers to doughnuts, pizza to french fries, and chicken to milkshakes. Fast-food restaurants were developing new ways to create food more and more quickly and cheaply.

That sounds like it would be a good thing. But these kinds of foods often have one things in common—they have lots of calories.

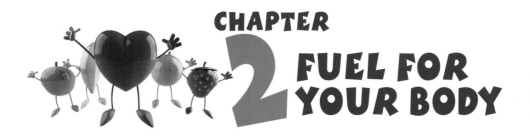

CHAPTER 2
FUEL FOR YOUR BODY

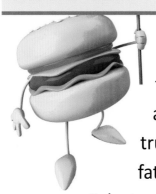

You've probably heard people talk about calories. Sometimes it may sound as though calories are bad things. After all, commercials are always making low-calorie foods sound as though they're healthier, and people who are on a diet will often count calories. It's true that too many calories can make us fat—but we also need calories.

Calories are a way to measure what's in the food we eat. We use inches and feet (or centimeters and meters) to measure how long or tall something is; we use pints and quarts (or liters) to measure liquids like milk and soda—and we use calories to measure how much *energy* is in a certain food.

What is **energy**?

Energy is the ability to be active, the power it takes to move your body.

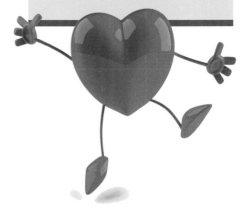

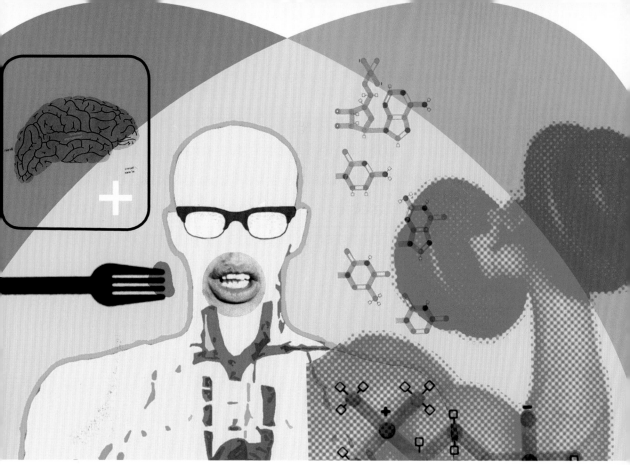

Food gives your body the fuel it needs to move, think, and carry on all the things it does inside your skin.

Each one of us needs a certain amount of calories every day to be healthy and have the energy we need for all the things we do in a day. Even sitting still takes a certain number of calories, but the more active we are, the more calories we need. People who are bigger, more active, or who are growing usually need more calories than smaller people, people who don't move around very much, and people who aren't growing.

BROCCOLI, ANYONE?

All foods have calories, whether it's cookies or carrots, lettuce or ice cream, but some foods have more calories than others. This means that if you ate a half cup of broccoli, you'd be getting about 12 calories—but if you ate a brownie, you'd be *consuming* more than ten times that amount of calories.

Per serving:

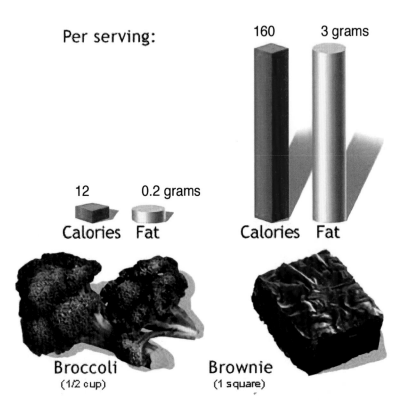

160   3 grams

12   0.2 grams

Calories   Fat   Calories   Fat

Broccoli   Brownie
(1/2 cup)   (1 square)

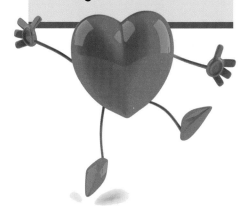

What does **consuming** mean?

It means eating or taking in.

DID YOU KNOW?

Most children between the ages of 5 and 12 need between 1,200 and 2,000 calories a day. Exactly how much they need will depend on how active they are, whether they're in the midst of a growth spurt, and how big they are.

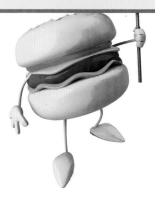

Both the broccoli and the brownie would take up about the same amount of room in your stomach, but there's a big difference in the number of calories! To take another example, a serving of carrot sticks (about a cup) would give you around 50 calories, while a serving of Oreos (3 cookies) would give you 210 calories. Or to look at it another way, if you ate a pound of lettuce, you would have eaten only about 80 calories (and you would have had to eat about 16 cups of lettuce!)—but if you ate a pound of chocolate chip cookies (about 10 cookies), you would have eaten 2,100 calories!

Of course, you might say you think the brownie and cookies taste better than the broccoli, carrots, and lettuce, but really, that's just a question of what you're used to eating.

CALORIES AS FUEL

Calories are the fuel your body needs to be active. They're like the gasoline that makes the engine run inside a car. Without gasoline, your car wouldn't be able to move out of the driveway—and without calories, you wouldn't have the energy to run around or do anything else. In fact, you wouldn't be able to be alive for very long!

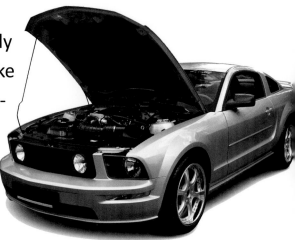

An engine burns gasoline to run—and your body burns calories.

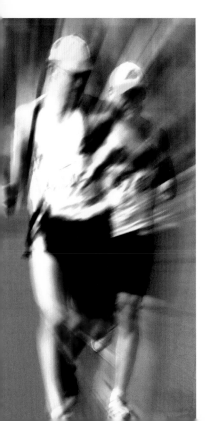

The chart on the next page shows the number of calories people of different weights burn while doing different exercises for an hour's time. You can see that the more you weigh, the more calories your body burns doing the same exercise.

Imagine that you're carry a 10-pound bag of sand—and then imagine that you're carrying a 100-pound bag. The heavier the weight, the more energy you need to move it. And the heavier your body is, the more energy it takes to move it around.

CALORIES AT WORK			
Activity (1 Hour)	130 lbs.	155 lbs.	190 lbs.
Aerobics (moderate impact)	354	422	518
Backpacking (general)	413	493	604
Badminton (social)	266	317	388
Basketball (game)	472	563	690
Bicycling (leisure, <10 mph)	236	281	345
Bicycling (stationary, moderate effort)	413	493	604
Billiards	148	176	216
Bowling	177	211	259
Circuit Training	472	563	690
Construction (outdoor)	325	387	474
Cooking	148	176	216
Flag Football	472	563	690
Football (competitive)	531	633	776
Frisbee (ultimate)	207	246	302
Golf (carrying clubs)	325	387	474
Golf (miniature)	177	211	259
Hiking (cross-country)	354	422	518
Hockey (ice or field)	472	563	690
Jogging (general)	413	493	604
Jumping Rope (moderate)	590	704	863
Kick-boxing/Karate/Judo	590	704	863
Lacrosse	472	563	690
Mowing the lawn (push mower)	325	387	474
Running (ten-minute mile)	590	704	863
Skateboarding	295	352	431
Skiing (x-country, moderate effort)	472	563	690
Skiing (downhill, moderate effort)	354	422	518
Soccer (competitive)	590	704	863
Softball or baseball (fast or slow pitch)	295	352	431
Volleyball (picnic, 6-9 members team)	177	211	259
Walking the dog (moderate pace)	207	246	302
Walking (briskly – 4 m.p.h.)	236	281	345

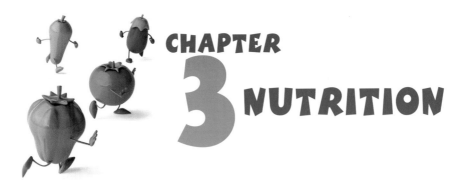

CHAPTER 3 NUTRITION

Since your body needs calories for fuel, you might think that the more calories a food has, the better it is for you. (And in that case, brownies and cookies would be better food choices than veggies.) But your body needs more than calories. It also needs *nutrition*.

CARBOHYDRATES

Carbohydrates, found in foods such as grain products, fruits, vegetables, and candy, are important sources of energy for your body. This means they're a good source of calories, but

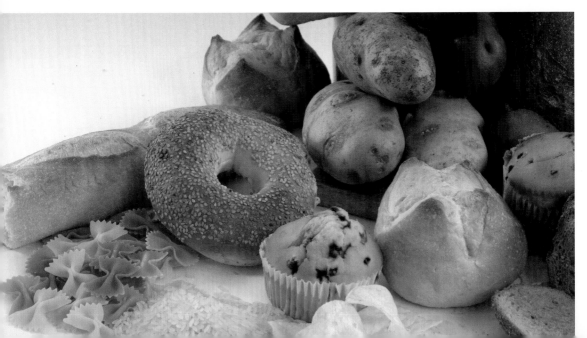

The fiber found in whole-grain breads is a complex carbohydrate that your body cannot break down, so it doesn't give you energy. Instead, it does another important job in your body—it keeps food moving through your intestines and out of your body.

they also contain other things your body needs. The healthiest carbohydrates are *complex* carbohydrates found in whole-grain foods like whole-wheat bread, long-grain brown rice, oatmeal, and many vegetables and fruits. Complex carbohydrates take a long time for your body to break down, so they give you energy for a longer period of time. Complex carbohydrates are also important because they are good sources of other nutrients, like vitamins and minerals, as well as fiber. Simple carbohydrates, on the other hand—like cookies, brownies, and candy—don't have many nutrients. And the energy they give you doesn't last very long.

Nutrition refers to the things in food that help your body live and grow.

Something that is **complex** has many parts.

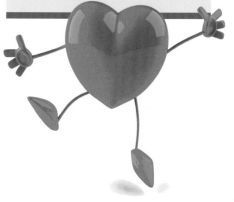

FATS

Fats are another nutrient. They've gotten a bad reputation, because people think that if you eat fats, you'll BE fat. But your body needs certain types of fats to be healthy.

Researchers have found that you need to get about 20 to 35 percent of your calories from fats. Each gram of fat you eat has nine calories. That's more than twice the amount of energy contained in a gram of carbohydrates or proteins, so it takes far fewer grams of fat to give you a lot of calories. That's one reason why eating too many fats can make you gain weight.

There are three kinds of fat—saturated (found in butter and meat), unsaturated (found in olive oil and vegetable oils),

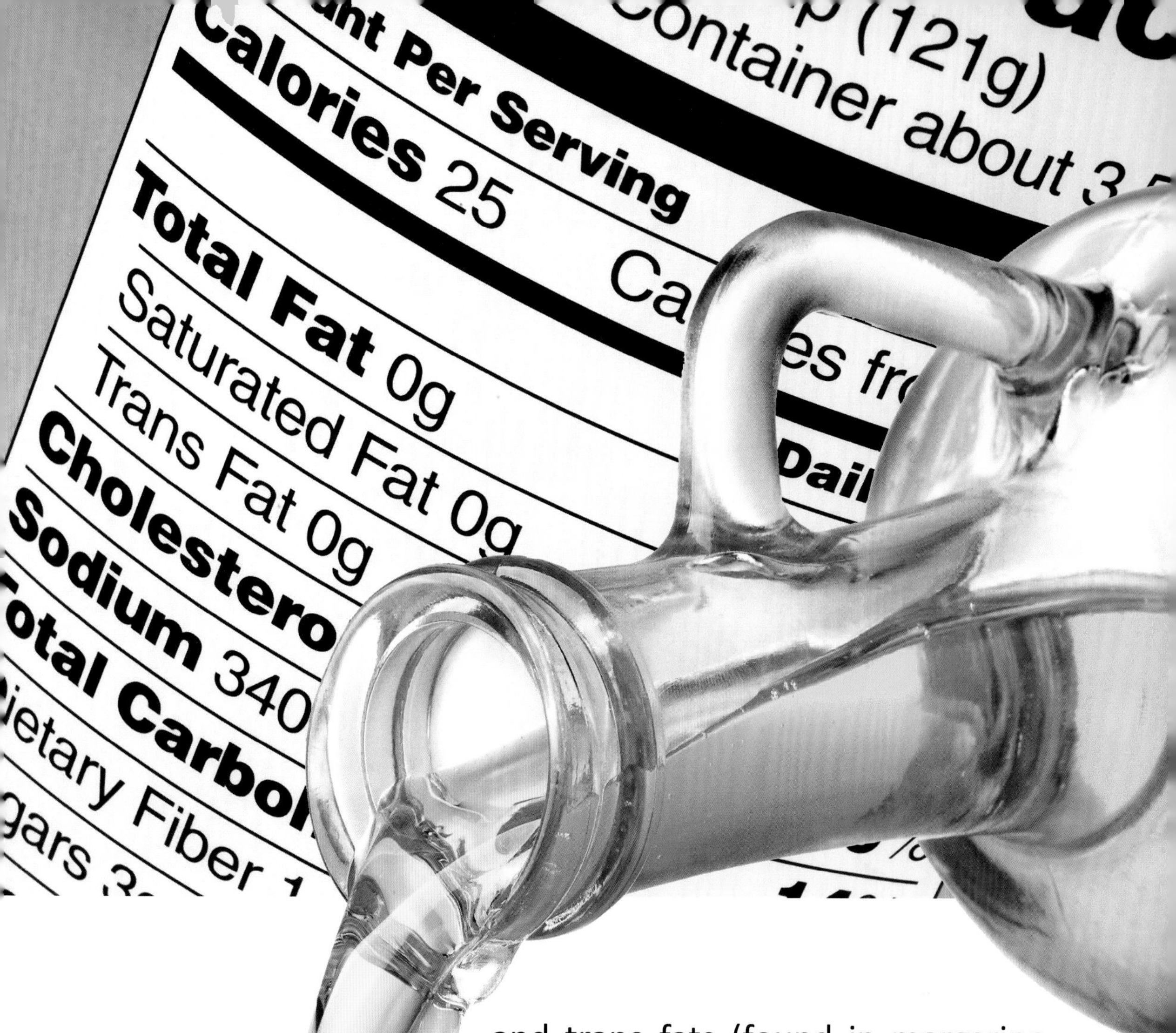

Calories Per Serving Container about 3.5 (121g)

Calories 25 Ca...

Total Fat 0g

Saturated Fat 0g

Trans Fat 0g

Cholestero...

Sodium 340

Total Carbo...

...ietary Fiber 1...

...gars 3...

and trans fats (found in margarine and shortening). Of these, unsaturated fats are best for you, and trans fats are worst. Many store-bought baked goods contain trans fats, so always check nutrition labels like the one shown here—and stay away from trans fats!

PROTEIN

Protein is another important nutrient. It's found in meat, eggs, and dairy products, as well as most grains, nuts, and legumes (like beans and peas). Protein is one of your body's most important building blocks. Without it, you could not build or repair muscles and other *tissues*. Protein also provides you with calories.

DIET MATH

To find out how much protein you need each day, multiply the number

The colorful ribbons and strings shown here represent strands of protein. Proteins are made up of long chains of chemicals strung together. Your muscles and your body's organs are all made of protein. Your body would not be able to heal scrapes and bruises without protein!

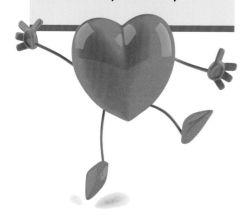

Tissues in your body are groups of cells that are alike and that work together to do the same job inside your body.

of calories you need by .10. Divide the answer by four (the number of calories in one gram of protein). This gives you the low-end of your necessary protein intake. Now multiply your calories by .35 and divide by four. This answer gives you the high-end for your protein intake. Here is an example for a person who needs 2,200 calories each day:

(2200 calories x .10) ÷ 4 calories per gram of protein = 55 grams

(2200 calories x .35) ÷ 4 calories per gram of protein = 192.5 grams

A person who needs 2,200 calories each day should eat approximately 55 to 192.5 grams of protein.

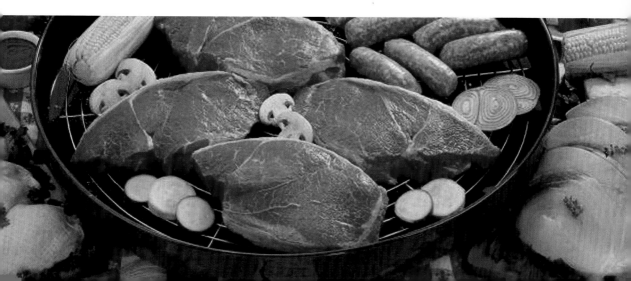

VITAMINS AND MINERALS

You also need vitamins and minerals to make your body work the way it should. Vitamins and minerals are often found in fruit and vegetables.

There are two kinds of vitamins—fat soluble and water soluble. The fat-soluble vitamins—A, D, E, and K—dissolve in fat and can be stored in your body. The water-soluble vitamins—C and the B vitamins (such as vitamins B6, B12, niacin, riboflavin, and folate)—need to be dissolved in water before your body can absorb them. Because of this, your body can't store these vitamins, so any vitamin C or B your body doesn't use leaves your body every day in your urine. That's why you need to get fresh supplies by eating fruits and vegetables every day.

Plants and animals make vitamins, but minerals come from the soil and water, and they are then absorbed by plants through their roots or eaten by animals.

Vitamins and minerals help you fight off germs and other things that might make you sick. Vitamins and minerals also help you grow, and they help all your cells and organs do their jobs.

DID YOU KNOW?

Your body needs larger amounts of some minerals, such as calcium to grow and stay healthy. Other minerals like chromium, copper, iodine, iron, selenium, and zinc are called trace minerals because you only need very small amounts of them each day.

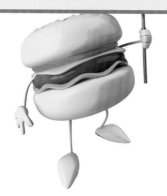

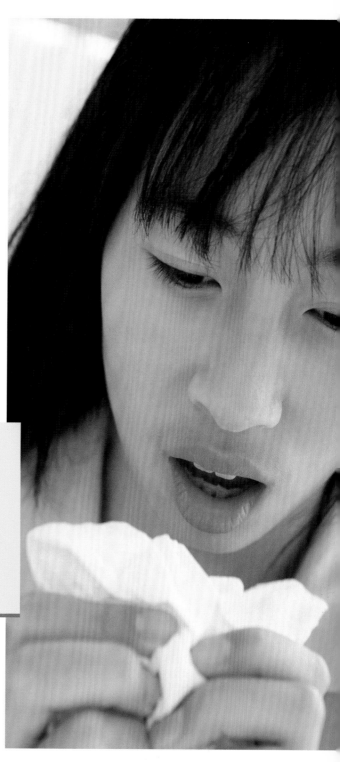

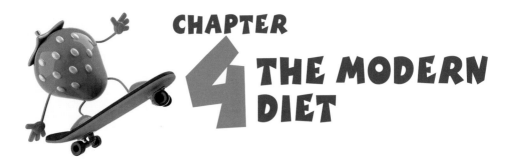

CHAPTER 4
THE MODERN DIET

Eating a variety of foods is the best way to get all the vitamins and minerals you need each day, as well as the right balance of carbohydrates, proteins, fats, and calories. Whole or un-processed foods—foods that are as close as possible to the way they grew naturally, without being frozen, canned, or packaged—are the best choices for getting the nutrients your body needs to stay healthy and grow properly.

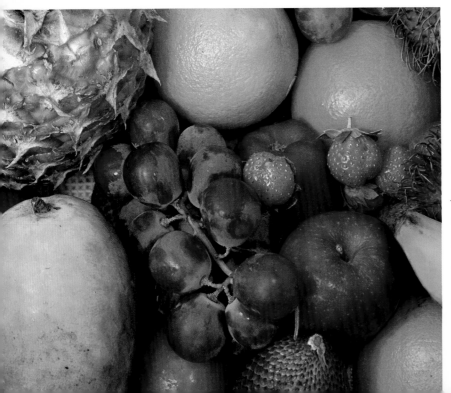

Fresh fruits that have never been processed—never cooked, canned, or frozen—have the most vitamins in them. This means they're the best for you.

But a lot of the foods we eat every day have been *processed*. This is true of almost ALL fast foods. The chicken nuggets shown here, for example, have come a long, long way since they were actual chickens! Along the way, the meat has lost a lot of the nutrients that make it good for you—and it has gained stuff that ISN'T good for you.

Food that has been **processed** has been canned or frozen. It has also often had chemicals added to it.

WHAT'S THE FAST-FOOD STORY?

Fast food has become a way of life for many of us. We swing through the drive-through on the way from school to baseball practice. We pick up take-out on busy nights when Mom doesn't have time to cook. We're always in a hurry, and fast foods help us cope with our busy lives.

But scientists who studied the foods served at fast-food restaurants discovered that these foods aren't that good for us. For one thing, they're high in fat, high in calories—and low in nutrition. Scientists also took a close look at the meat used in fast food—the chicken and beef—and they found out some yucky things! The chemicals in the meat told them that the animals had been fed corn, which makes them as fat as possible in as short a time as possible, and that they had been raised in a very small space where their own manure got mixed with their food. This means that the meat isn't as healthy for us to eat, but it also means that the animals weren't living in very good conditions.

DID YOU KNOW?

Cows and chickens that are allowed to wander around in fields eating grass and other natural foods turn into meat that is healthier for people to eat.

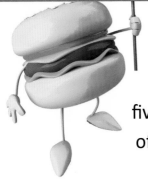

In order to get the nutrition our bodies need to be healthy, we need to eat at least five servings of vegetables and five servings of fruit every day. But most fast foods don't contain either fruits or vegetables. Some fast-food restaurants are trying to change, though, by offering more salads and fruit snacks. If your family eats often at fast-food restaurants, pay attention to what you're eating. This chart shows you the calories, fat, and other nutritional values for common fast foods.

Food	Serving size (g.)	Calories	Total Fat (g.)	Sat. Fat (g.)	Chol. (mg)	Sodium (mg)	Carb. (g)	Fiber (g)	Sugar (g)	Protein (g)
McDonald's										
Big Mac ®	219	600	33	11	85	1050	50	4	8	25
Chicken McNuggets® (6 piece)	96	250	15	3	35	670	15	0	0	15
Grilled Chicken Bacon Ranch Salad (w/2 oz. Ranch dressing)	288	260	25	7	105	1460	18	3	7	32
Med. Fries	114	350	17	3	0	220	44	4	0	5
Burger King										
Original WHOPPER ®	291	700	42	13	85	1020	52	4	8	31
Original Chicken Sandwich	204	560	28	6	60	1270	52	3	5	25
Fire-Grilled Shrimp Garden Salad (w/2 oz. Sweet Onion Vinaigrette)	406	300	18	4	120	1860	21	3	13	21
Med. Onion Rings	91	320	16	4	0	460	40	3	5	4
Subway										
6" Sweet Onion Chicken Teriyaki Sandwich	271	370	5	1.5	50	1090	59	5	9	26
6" Meatball Marinara	288	500	22	11	45	1180	52	5	9	23
Classic Club Salad (w/1 packet Kraft Fat Free Italian dressing)	487	425	21	10	210	2540	20	4	9	38
Brown and Wild Rice w/ Chicken Soup	240	190	11	4.5	20	990	17	2	3	6
Pizza Hut										
1 Cheese Breadstick	67	200	10	3.5	15	340	21	1	4	7
12" Supreme Medium Pan Pizza (1 slice)	127	320	16	6	25	650		2	30	13
14" Sausage Lover's Stuffed Crust Pizza (! Slice)	162	430	19	9	50	1130	43	3	9	19
12" Ham, Red Onion, and Mushroom Fit 'N Delicious (1 Slice)	101	160	4.5	2	15	470	22	2	6	8
Taco Bell										
Fresco Style Soft Beef Taco	113	190	8	3	20	630	22	3	3	9
Bean Burrito	198	370	10	3.5	10	1200	55	8	4	14
Chicken Chalupa Baja	153	400	24	6	40	690	30	2	4	17
Nachos Supreme	195	450	26	9	35	800	42	7	4	13

PORTION SIZES

There are a few things wrong with the modern diet. One is that we eat too much processed and fast foods. And another problem is the size of our servings.

For example, if you go to a movie, does your family order a tub of popcorn? Twenty years ago a family-size portion of popcorn was about 5 cups, and had 270 calories— but that tub of popcorn you're eating today holds about 11.5 cups of popcorn, and it gives you 630 calories. And do you eat bagels for breakfast? Well, twenty years ago, the average bagel was 3 inches wide and had 140 calories. Today it's more than 5 inches wide, and it will give you 350 calories. And if you're going through the drive-thru at the fast-food restaurant, the burgers you buy are two to five times larger than the ones your parents were eating twenty years ago—and they have at least twice as many calories.

So what do you think that means for our weight? Well, it's not just our portion sizes that have been *expanding*—so have our waistlines! People tend to eat whatever is put before them. And we also often think that bigger is better. But when it comes to food, that's not true!

Something that is **expanding** is getting bigger and bigger.

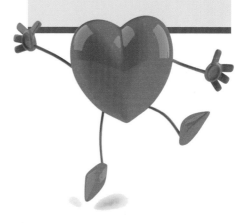

And It's not just food portions that have been growing bigger over the years. Plate, bowl, and cup sizes have gotten bigger as well. In the early 1990s, the standard size of a dinner plate increased from 10 to 12 inches; cup and bowl sizes also got bigger. You might think that wouldn't matter, but scientists have found that people tend to fill up their plates, no matter how big they are. Larger eating containers can make people eat more.

There are plenty of other examples of our expanding portions, but junk foods are some of the worst. Candy bars are bigger today than they used

DID YOU KNOW?

A can of Coke contains about 10 teaspoons of sugar. Sugar is high in calories, low in nutrition—and it's bad for your teeth!

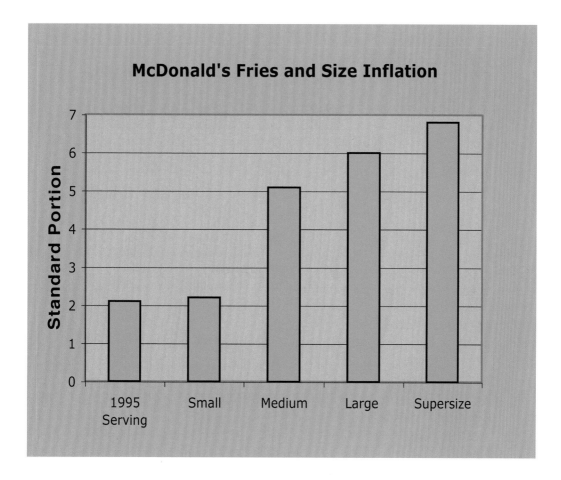

McDonald's Fries and Size Inflation

to be. And take a look at soft-drink bottles. When your parents were your age, a bottle of Coke held 8 ounces and contained 97 calories. It wasn't exactly a healthy beverage even then—but at least it wasn't the wopping 20-ounce bottle it is today, containing 242 calories. We feel like we're getting more for our money when we buy these larger sizes—but really we're just getting fatter for our money!

5 MAKE A CHANGE FOR THE BETTER!

DID YOU KNOW?

Food isn't the only thing your body needs to be healthy. You also need to drink plenty of water every day. Your body is actually made mostly of water, and it needs water in order to be healthy and work the way it's supposed to.

Have you ever heard someone say, "You are what you eat"? What they mean is that the food you eat gets broken down and tuned into your body's cells. If you eat the nutrients you need—carbohydrates, protein, vitamins, minerals, and the right kind of fats—your body will be able to grow and be strong and healthy. But if you don't eat the nutrients your body needs, your body will be more likely to get sick. It may not grow normally. And if you eat too many calories, more than your body needs for fuel, you will store those calories as fat—and you'll end up overweight or obese.

So should you go on a diet tomorrow? No! *Experts* say that dieting really isn't the best way to lose weight or be healthy. People may lose weight on a diet, but they also may not get the nutrients they need. And after a while, most people feel start feeling frustrated—and HUNGRY! Sooner or later, they go back to eating the way they did before. Sometimes they eat even more than they did before.

The best way to lose weight and be healthy is to change the way you think about food. Make a change for the better!

> **Experts** are people who know a lot about a certain thing because they've studied it and worked with it a lot.

STOP BELIEVING COMMERCIALS!

You're probably used to seeing commercials on television. You may think some of them are annoying, and you may like others. Some may make you laugh. But whatever you think, those commercials are shaping the way you think about food.

The companies that make junk food, sugary cereals, and juice boxes know that if kids like what they make, the kids will ask their parents to buy these products. The more these companies sell, the more money they make. So these companies put lots of commericals on television during kids' shows.

These commercials are aimed right at you! They're made to convince you that you NEED a candy bar or a certain kind of cereal or a special packaged kids' meal.

Every year, companies spend $1 billion on ads and com-

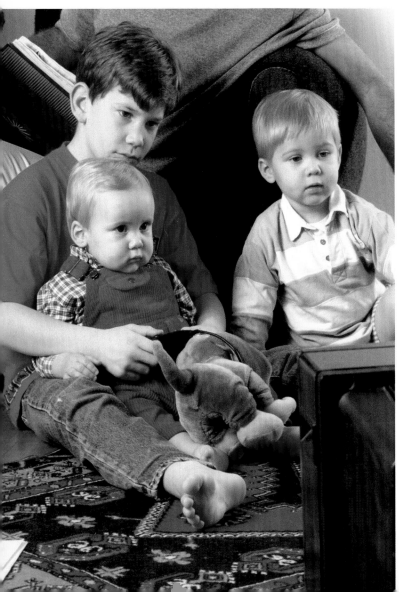

Children between the ages of 2 and 17 watch about 18,000 hours of television in a year. That's more time than they spend in school!

mercials that are meant for children. Even very young children watch television, and the more times they see the same message, the more likely they are to believe it. So if you hear over and over that Yummy Sweeties are delicious and fun and will make you happy, then you end up believing that you really, really want to eat Yummy Sweeties. You tell your parents to please, please, PLEASE buy you Yummy Sweeties. You point them out to your dad when you go grocery shopping, you beg your mom to give them to you if you clean your room, you persuade your grandma to keep them on hand for you as a special treat. Pretty soon Yummy Sweeties are one of your favorite foods, and you can't imagine living without them.

MAKE UP YOUR MIND FOR YOURSELF!

So if you want to be healthier, stop listening to the messages on TV commericals. Instead, learn about what you need to do to have a healthier diet. Talk about it with your family and friends. The more people think about eating healthier and talk about it, the more people—and the entire world—will begin to change, little by little.

Moderation means not too much and not too little.

Don't just accept what goes on around you and follow along blindly. Ask questions. Learn about what a healthy lifestyle looks like. Find out about healthier ways to eat. You may be still a kid, but you can make up your own mind to take care of your body better and keep it healthier. Try new foods. Eat more carrots—and fewer cookies!

Does this mean you have to give up foods like potato chips, candy bars, and cookies forever? No, it's okay to have these foods once in a while. Just don't eat too many of them. Practice *moderation*!

Try to eat a balanced diet that has lots of different kinds of foods, so you get all the nutrients you need.

TAKE AN HONEST LOOK AT YOURSELF

You may not be overweight or obese now. But as you get older, you might gain weight. To find out if you're likely to have a problem with your weight as you get older, answer the following questions as honestly as you can:

1. Do you usually take less than twenty minutes to eat a meal?
2. After finishing your meal, do you still feel hungry?
3. When you sit down to eat, do you eat everything put in front of you no matter how big the portion size?
4. Does your diet include large amounts of high-sugar or high-fat foods?
5. Do you exercise at least three days each week?
6. Do you eat a balanced diet each and every day?

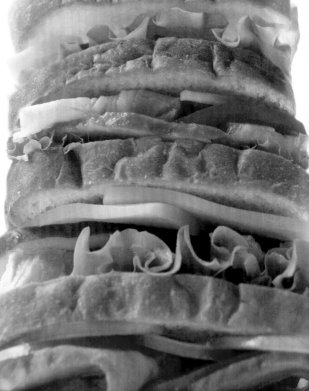

If you answered yes to the first three questions or no to questions 5 and 6, you may find that you gain weight as you get older. But don't wait till you have a problem! The more weight you have to lose, the

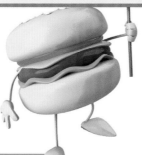

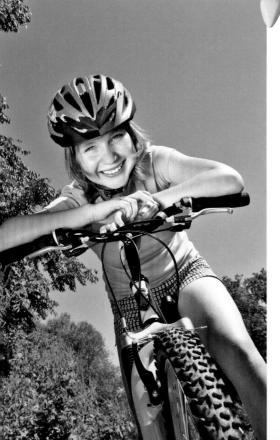

harder it is to do. Do what you can to change your lifestyle now.

TAKE ACTION!

The best way to lose weight, experts tell us, is to change the way you live. Form new habits. This isn't easy—but new ways of living become easier to do the more we do them. Learn to take care of your body every day.

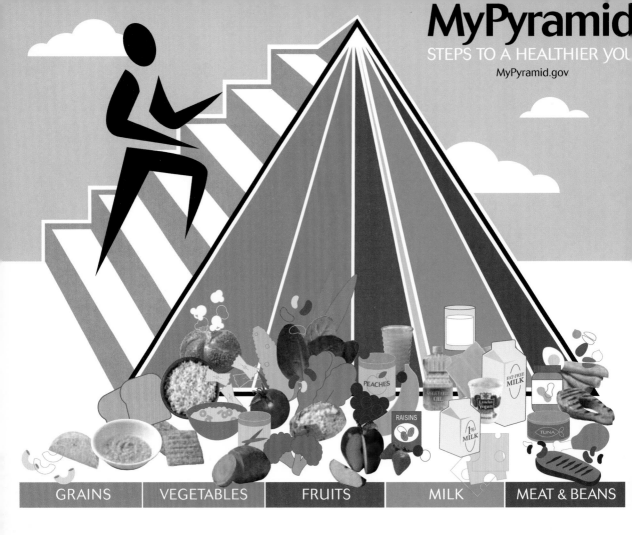

MyPyramid
STEPS TO A HEALTHIER YOU
MyPyramid.gov

| GRAINS | VEGETABLES | FRUITS | MILK | MEAT & BEANS |

CHANGING WHAT YOU EAT

Don't expect to change all at once. Every day, though, try to do something that's good for your body by eating fresh vegetables and fruits. Choose whole-grain bread instead of white bread. Drink water or milk instead of soda or juice. Big changes happen a little at a time!

Scientists have discovered the best combination of foods your body needs to be healthy. A diagram of this combination looks like a pyramid, with the foods you need to eat more at the

DID YOU KNOW?

A balanced diet is one that includes all the food groups shown on the food pyramid. In other words, have foods from every color, every day.

bottom, and the foods you need to eat less at the top. The U.S. Department of Agriculture, the part of the American government that deals with food, farming, and nutrition, has created a picture called "MyPyramid" to help you understand better how much and what kinds of foods you need to eat in order to be healthy.

It's okay to eat cookies sometimes. Just be sure to eat some carrots too!

You can see the bands on MyPyramid start out wider and get thinner as they go up. That's to show you that not all foods are the same, even within a healthy food group like fruit. For instance, apple pie would be in the thin part of the fruit band because it has a lot of added sugar and fat. A whole apple would be down in the wide part because you can eat more of those in a healthy diet.

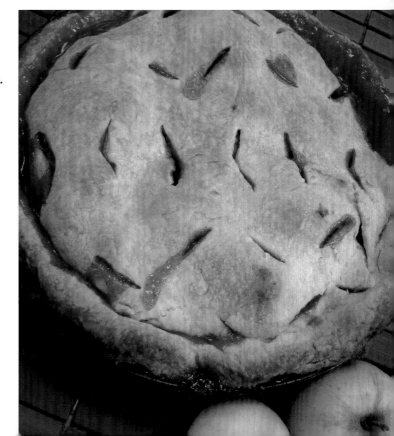

READ MORE ABOUT IT

Bean, Anita. *Awesome Foods for Active Kids: The ABCs of Eating for Energy and Health*. Alameda, Calif.: Hunter House, 2006.

Dolgoff, Joanna. *Red Light, Green Light, Eat Right: The Food Solution That Lets Kids Be Kids*. Emmaus, Penn.: Rodale, 2009.

Gaesser, Glenn. *Big Fat Lies: The Truth About Your Weight and Your Health.* Carlsbad, Calif.: Gürze Books, 2002.

Johnson, Susan and Laurel Mellin. *Just for Kids!* (Obesity Prevention Workbook). San Anselmo, Calif.: Balboa Publishing, 2002.

Vos, Miriam B. *The No-Diet Obesity Solution for Kids*. Bethesda, Md.: AGA Institute, 2009.

Zinczenko, David and Matt Goulding. *Eat This Not That! For Kids!* Emmaus, Penn.: Rodale, 2008.

FIND OUT MORE ON THE INTERNET

The Learning Center
www.hebs.scot.nhs.uk/learningcentre/obesity/intro/index.cfm

MyPyramid Blast Off Game
www.mypyramid.gov/kids/kids_game.html

Small Step Kids
www.smallstep.gov/kids/html/games_and_activities.html

INDEX

PICTURE CREDITS

ABOUT THE AUTHOR

Helen Thompson lives in upstate New York. She worked first as a social worker and then became a teacher as her second career. She has taught health topics to kids in grades six through eight, and she has attended workshops in nutrition and fitness. Although she has never been an athlete, she enjoys hiking regularly, and works hard to maintain a high-fiber, low-fat diet.